All Yo ... t

Hair Care

Editorial Board

Meenakshi Sinha

Reena Rajgopal

Suchismita Banerjee

New Dawn

NEW DAWN
An imprint of Sterling Publishers (P) Ltd.
L-10, Green Park Extension, New Delhi-110016
Ph.: 6191784, 6191785, 6191023 Fax: 91-11-6190028
E-mail: ghai@nde.vsnl.net.in
Internet: http://www.sterlingpublishers.com

All You Wanted to Know About - Hair Care

ISBN 81 207 2353 8

Published by Sterling Publishers Pvt. Ltd., New Delhi-110016.
Lasertypeset by Vikas Compographics, New Delhi-110029.
Printed at Shagun Composer New Delhi-110029.

Contents

Preface

This book will prove to be of great help to those who wish to have beautiful, healthy hair. Some people are lucky enough to be born with amazingly beautiful hair while those who are not, can help themselves with the information provided in this book.

Introduction

Every one longs for beautiful hair that is healthy, lustrous and easy to maintain. The first step towards this goal would be to choose the right hair care product that suits your hair. Different types of hair need different hair-care products. The use of wrong hair care products can prove detrimental to the hair.

So, take care of your hair in much the same way as you take care of your skin. Use the right hair care products and follow an effective hair care regimen involving cleaning, toning and conditioning routines, carried out with religious regularity.

This book will inform you about the routines that you need to follow and the treatment that you need to take to overcome your hair problems.

The Structure and Growth of Hair

Shape of Hair

Human hair is remarkable, for it adds so much to one's good looks and personality. Different people have different kinds of hair — it can be coarse, medium or fine; curly, wavy or straight; and thick, thin or in-between. It all depends on the inherent structure and the nourishment provided to the hair.

A part of each hair extends below the surface of the skin. This part lies

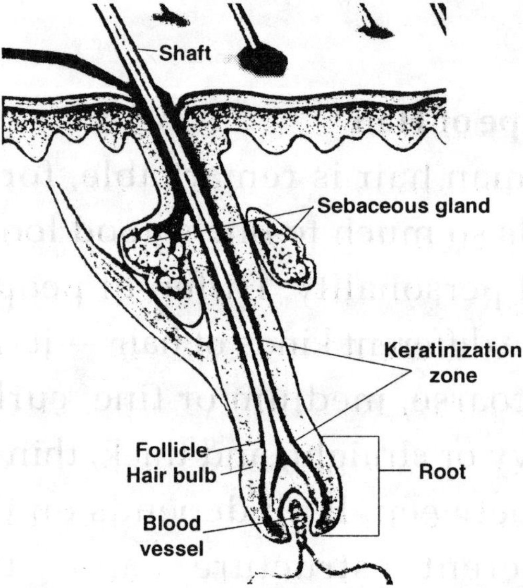

The Structure of Hair

in a bag-like structure called the follicle. The end of the hair, called the *bulb* is the only living part of a hair. It lies in the dermis or the subcutaneous tissue. The cells of the bulb divide rapidly and account for the growth of a hair.

Each hair grows, then rests, then drops out or is pushed out by new hair. Each follicle operates on its own timetable. Usually ninety per cent of the hair on your head grow at one time. The other ten per cent rest. A hair's life cycle can last anywhere from two to six years. The longer the growing stage, the longer is the hair.

Though each hair strand looks like a single fibre, it is however made up of three distinct layers: the cuticle, the cortex and the medulla.

The diagram shows the three layers of dead cells that constitute a hair strand:

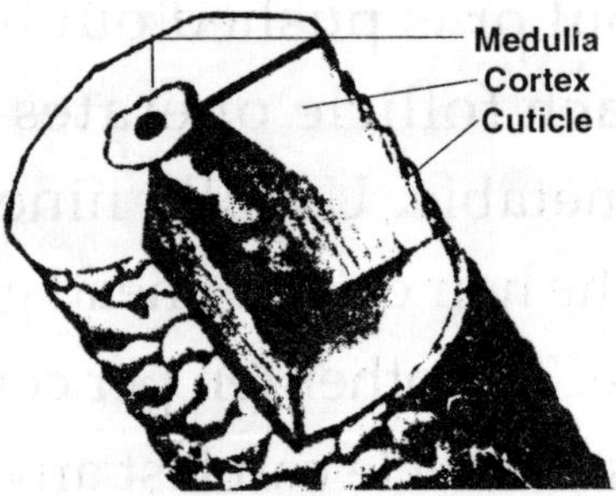

The Three Layers of a Hair Strand

Cuticle

- It is the outermost layer.
- It provides protection from the external elements.
- It has tiny transparent scales which overlap one another and contribute to the shine.
- When these scales wear away, the hair loses its natural lustre and looks dull and rough.
- When the cuticle breaks and dislodges at the end of the hair, it results in split ends.
- Improper care and frequent use of harsh chemicals on the hair damage the cuticle.

Cortex

- It is the middle layer.
- It consists of fibres twisted together.
- Its composition affects the colour, strength, elasticity, growth, width and texture of the hair.

Medulla

- It is the innermost layer.
- It is made up of soft keratin.
- It does not have any significant role to play.

On an average, hair grows at the rate of about 2.5 cms a month. The growth of hair in the follicles occurs in cycles. In each cycle, a follicle goes through a growth phase and a resting phase.

A hair stops growing during every resting phase, and is known as a *club hair*. The club hair remains in the resting follicle until the next growing phase. During the growing phase, the club hair is shed as a new hair grows and pushes it out of the follicle.

The length of hair depends on the length of the growing phase of the follicle. The follicles in the human scalp are active for two or six years and then they rest for about three months.

The most effective period of hair growth in women is between fifteen and forty years, when they produce maximum estrogen. Hair never stops growing — the rate at which it grows changes with biological, and environmental changes.

Many factors affect the growth of hair. They include age, diet, general health, and changes in the weather. For example, hair grows faster in children than in adults, and it grows faster in summer than during any other season.

Cutting or shaving hair on any part of the body does not have any effect on the future growth or texture of the hair.

Hair Colour

Your hair colour is set at birth. It is inherited and determined by a pigment called melanin.

The darker your hair is, the more melanin it contains. As you might guess, blonde hair has very little melanin and grey hair has no melanin at all.

Whether or not your hair will turn grey in the future depends mostly on your genes and how much melanin your body makes. Most people's hair gradually becomes grey or white as they grow older, because the pigment cells producing melanin become inactive, resulting in white hair.

This could also happen because of an illness, sudden shock, some internal disorder or your genetic make-up.

What makes Hair Curly?

The shape of your hair follicles determines whether you have straight, wavy or curly hair.

- Straight hair usually grows from a round hair shaft.
- Wavy hair tends to grow from an oval shaft.
- Curly hair grows from a nearly flat shaft.

What is Healthy Hair?

All of us want our hair to be healthy. However, there is no one definition of healthy hair. Due to the different composition of each person's hair, factors which affect its health are different.

You can decide whether your hair is healthy or not based upon some of these factors.

Is your hair –

- Thick and Dense?
- Fine and silky?
- Shiny and glossy?

- Easy to style?
- Having Body and Bounce?
- Having good and regular growth?

Your hair is healthy, if your answers to these questions are in the affirmative.

Diet and Hair

How your hair looks, depends a great deal on your diet. Remember, hair is nourished from the inside. A well-balanced, nutritious diet will work wonders for your hair.

Iron deficiency causes maximum damage to the hair by lowering the haemoglobin level, which in turn reduces the oxygen-carrying capacity of the blood. Oxygen deficiency weakens the hair follicles, leading to dryness of the scalp and hair loss.

Proteins and calcium are extremely important for tissues. Any deficiency of either proteins or calcium can permanently damage your hair, therefore a diet rich in protein and calcium is recommended.

Soyabean, as we all know is one of the richest sources of proteins — and hence is good for hair. But undigested soyabean is harmful, hence it is essential to eat only the requisite amount of soyabean.

Milk is a rich source of calcium and, therefore, essential for healthy hair. All milk products too are good for hair.

Minerals and vitamin supplements like zinc, vitamin B, etc., are also essential for the body.

Too much of fat-soluble vitamins like A, D, E or K can damage your liver for they do not get flushed out; instead they are stored in the body. But Vitamin B, being water soluble, is absorbed in required quantities and the rest is expelled from the body.

Yeast is a rich source of vitamin B, and hence people suffering from various hair-disorders should include yeast in their diet.

Curd (yogurt) is very good for hair, not only through diet but also through external application. It is easily digestible and is an excellent source of vitamin B; it also contains a type of bacteria which is very good for skin and hair.

Iodine is another element which is essential for healthy hair. Most of us have noticed that people living in coastal areas have thick hair. The credit goes to iodine, which is present in fish.

Fruits like plums and vegetables like brinjal are also rich in iodine.

Care for Different Types of Hair

Types of Hair

Before we get down to hair care, it is important to determine what kind of hair you have. Different types of hair need different hair care products. The use of wrong products is detrimental to the hair.

Always use products made by reputed companies, check the date of manufacturing and never use products more than a year old.

Dry Hair

- The lack of sebum and oil causes dry hair.
- Flakiness of the scalp and dandruff are a direct result of dryness.
- If these is dryness the hair looks limp, tends to look thin and rough, becomes less elastic, loses its body and bounce.
- Dry hair is susceptible to breakage and damage.

Tips for Care of Dry Hair

- Your hair care routine should aim at replenishing the oil and the moisture in your hair, as excessive dryness can cause your hair to become brittle.
- Hair can also become dry due to rigorous cleansing routines and dry toning exercises. Condition your hair properly – for it restores and corrects the imbalance of moisture and oil in your hair.

- Use a good hair oil to massage your hair. It is a good idea to steam the scalp before a hot oil massage. With fingers planted firmly on the head, work the fingers in small, circular strokes, first clockwise and then anti-clockwise, to massage your scalp.
- If the hair is extremely dry, rub a little oil right into the roots before steaming. This is even more beneficial, as the subsequent steaming and a second massage with oil encourages better and deeper absorption.

- Frequent shampooing is harmful — never use a strong shampoo.
- Never comb, brush or massage vigorously.

Normal Hair

- The hair is healthy, shiny and silky without over-dry ends or over-oily roots.
- It has a good body and bounce.
- It is easy to cope with and care for normal hair.

Tips for Care of Normal Hair

- To maintain the balance of neither too oily nor too dry, condition your hair regularly.
- Use a good hair oil to massage your hair.

- Frequent shampooing is harmful —never use a strong shampoo.
- Never comb, brush or massage vigorously.

Oily Hair

- When the oil (sebaceous) glands in the scalp secrete excess oil, it travels down the hair shaft, causing excessive oiliness of the scalp and hair.
- Oily hair therefore appears lanky, dark and coarse.

Tips for Care of Oily Hair

- The hair care routine should aim at removing the excess oil and the dead skin cells which clog up and suffocate the hair follicles in the scalp.

- Regular cleansing helps wash away the excess oil from your hair and scalp and removes the dead skin cells.
- Wash your hair every third or fourth day, with a good quality herbal shampoo.
- Toning helps you to keep your hair healthy.
- Toning of the scalp and hair is achieved by gently massaging the head with your fingers, which helps in stimulating and invigorating the blood circulation required for the healthy growth of hair.

- Do not use hair oil, instead, use a good quality toning lotion.
- Excessive oiliness, when neglected, often leads to falling hair and premature baldness in men. So it should not be neglected, for prevention is always better than cure.

Hair Brushes and Combs

Brushes and combs are essential elements for hair care. Avoid sharing your hair brushes, clean them properly and change them whenever they are worn out.

Using the right kind of hair brush for your hair is essential, for the wrong kind could damage your hair permanently.

You should have two hair brushes in your hair kit:

- An oval, medium-sized brush for general grooming and adding volume to your style.

- A round brush to de-tangle your hair and to straighten it.

It is better to use a brush with natural bristles, for it works more gently on your hair and scalp.

If you are using a plastic comb, make sure that it is gentle and does not damage the scalp.

Another point to remember – clean your hair brush on a regular basis. Every time you wash your hair – give your hair brush a wash too.

A dirt-clogged hair brush does not glide smoothly through the hair, thereby breaking the hair and damaging the scalp.

To clean a hair brush/comb, ensure that all the loose hair is removed before soaking it in lukewarm water. Then after five minutes brush out all the excess dirt, rinse well with water (an antiseptic could also be used) and leave it to dry naturally.

Disorders of the Hair and Scalp

Like human beings, hair also has a life-cycle but unlike human beings, each hair survives only for about 4-5 years, after which the hair falls off from the head and a new hair begins to grow in its place. Every hair that grows must fall out one day. New hair will grow at the same place, after some time.

There is a natural balance between the rate at which the hair falls and the rate at which new hair grows. Any disturbance in this balance can result in an emotionally discomfiting condition of either an excess fallout of hair or hairiness all over the body. However, if your hair is shedding faster than the normal rate, you may have a 'falling hair' problem.

Hair Loss

The various causes of excessive hair loss are:

Heredity

Your body structure is influenced to a great deal by the genes that you have inherited. The problems concerning hair loss are therefore, many a time, passed on from parents to their children.

Trauma and Stress

Physical stress on the hair, caused by tying the hair too tightly can result in spot baldness due to the prolonged and continuous pull-like pressure on the hair. A trauma, sudden shock or a severe blow can also cause spot baldness where the blow is received.

Local Scalp Infection

Bacterial, viral or fungal infections can also cause spot baldness.

Diseases

Internal disorders and infections which cause high fever such as flu, pneumonia and typhoid are often accompanied by excessive hair loss.

Chemicals or Drugs

Certain antibiotics and other strong drugs can sometimes lead to hair loss. Chemical therapies given in serious diseases such as cancer also causes hair loss.

Emotional or Environmental Stress

People who are unable to cope with the pressure of life, constantly worry about the problems at the work place or home. They have most of their emotional conflicts unresolved and hence are easy victims to excess hair loss. Because of accumulated tensions in the mind, the muscles in the scalp and neck constrict. The blood circulation is thereby impeded, resulting in the suffocation of the hair cells, which in turn results in their dying and falling off.

Hormonal Imbalances and Hair Loss

Hormonal imbalances are the primary cause of serious hair loss in women. Pregnancy, contraception through birth control pills, and menopause, are the common conditions that induce hormonal changes.

Pregnancy

Generally, the hair condition improves during pregnancy as the endocrine glands function at their peak. The hair loss occurs only after the birth of the baby. This happens due to irregularity in the functioning of the thyroid glands. The hair loss can be attributed to the change in life style – the new unaccustomed life with the baby. The hair loss begins four months after delivery and continues for about two months.

On an average 25-30 strands of hair are shed daily and new ones grow to replace them. Baldness develops when the new hair stops growing for some reason.

Baldness

Baldness or *alopecia* is the partial or total absence of hair on the scalp. It occurs when the follicles on the scalp die and fail to produce new hair. Heredity is the most common cause of baldness.

However, other factors, including scalp infections and reactions to drugs or radiation can also cause baldness.

Some kinds of baldness involve only a thinning of the hair or loss of hair from a small area on the scalp

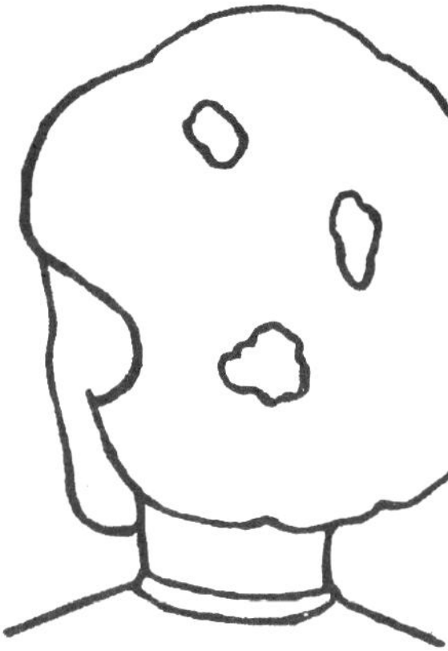

Pattern Baldness

— leaving the hair on the scalp in uneven patches.

The most common type of baldness, is called *male pattern baldness,* in which a man loses much, or all of his hair from the top of his head. Heredity is the most common cause of this kind of baldness.

A few women face the condition known as *female pattern baldness* which involves thinning of hair but not complete baldness. Pattern baldness cannot be cured.

However, many types of baldness are temporary, and in such cases, normal hair growth can be restored. It is essential to consult a dermatologist for treatment.

Medicated hair tonics and ointments are prescribed to control infection and restore health to the hair. The problem of hair loss is checked and hair growth recurs.

It is essential to treat hair gently. When there is a problem of hair loss, hair becomes even more fragile than usual. Hence it becomes essential not to comb, brush or massage the hair vigorously.

Sometimes, hair loss begins with the loss of essential nutrients and minerals from your scalp, leaving you with damaged, broken hair and finally, thin hair. Your hair's health can be restored by using 'Trichosaccharide', a natural biological nutrient discovered and patented in Italy.

Trichosaccharide, when in contact with the connective tissue of your scalp, increases the sulphur content of the hair follicles, promotes keratin synthesis, improves microcirculation and finally makes nutritive substances available to the hair bulb. This action replenishes your thinning hair and gives you thicker and healthier hair in weeks.

Dandruff

Dandruff is the single most common problem and the number one enemy of healthy hair. It is the result of excessive flaking of dead skin cells in your scalp.

Dandruff results when oil and loose cells cling to each other and stick to the scalp.

There are two forms of dandruff—oily and dry. Dry dandruff is most common and appears as loose white flakes, and the scalp itches a great deal. Oily

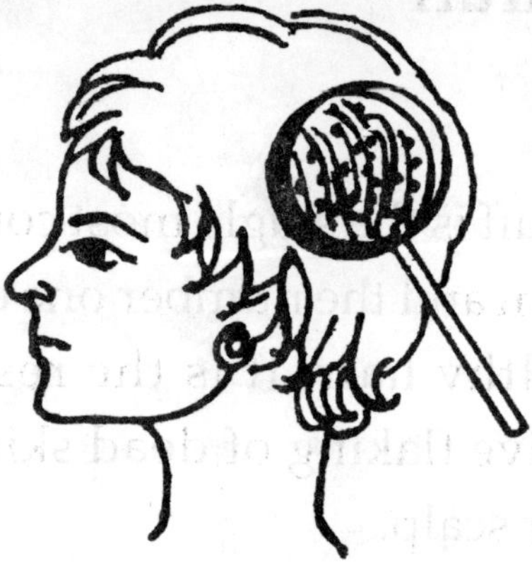

Dandruff

dandruff is sticky and yellow in colour, and the scalp smells bad with oily dandruff. The oily form is found most among adolescents and adults with an excessively oily skin and scalp.

Causes of Dandruff

Dandruff is generally caused by an excessive growth of microbes (bacteria) on the scalp. This could be the result of a faulty diet, emotional tension and stress, hormonal disturbances, infection due to disease, injury to the scalp, unwise or excessive use of hair cosmetics and dry weather.

Androgens (male hormones) which cause baldness in men are also responsible for greasy hair and dandruff.

The actual cause of dandruff is a mystery even for doctors, and most people face this problem at some time. Dandruff does not cause permanent baldness, though in extreme cases it might result in severe hair-loss.

How to Get Rid of Dandruff ?

The first step is to keep the hair clean. Wash your hair and scalp frequently: it could be daily or every other day depending upon how stubborn your dandruff is. Use a good anti-dandruff shampoo.

Massaging and brushing your hair frequently is also extremely helpful in treating dandruff. They invigorate the blood circulation to the scalp, promote oil secretion and dislodge the dead skin cells sticking to your scalp.

Avoid hair sprays and lotions that can build up on your hair. Use an anti-dandruff or medicated shampoo, containing zinc pyrithione or selenium sulphide or corticosteroid hormones. To start with, use it once a week and as the dandruff condition improves, reduce the usage to once a month.

If the situation persists, a dermatologist should be consulted.

Treatment with herbal extracts has been found to be extremely effective.

Herbs like henna, *shikakai, reetha,* and *amla* are antiseptic ingredients provided by nature and have a powerful cleansing action, without any harmful effects like those of detergents.

Pure coconut oil or olive oil can be heated and applied on the scalp. It should be left overnight. Next day, apply the juice of a lemon on your scalp. Shampoo your hair after an hour. This is a good treatment for dandruff.

Applying henna on the hair also helps in controlling dandruff.

Where dandruff is concerned, it is vital to keep the hair, combs, towels and pillow cases absolutely clean, as there are chances of re-infection.

Premature Greying of Hair

Grey hair on one's head does not necessarily mean growing older – for it could even take place in your twenties.

Grey hair is caused due to malfunctioning of melanin-producing cells. These specialized cells stop producing melanin in requisite quantities and hence due to its absence, the hair looks grey.

Amla has hair-darkening properties and therefore to delay or prevent greying of hair, use amla based hair oils and shampoo.

Another tip to prevent greying of hair is to include a teaspoon of curry leaf chutney in your diet every day.

Premature greying of hair is a genetic disorder and the greying of hair with age is controlled by genes, hence there is no cure for it. However you can colour your hair to make it beautiful and vibrant again.

To colour your hair, you could either use a chemical or a natural dye. The advantage of using a natural dye is that it is completely safe.

Henna is probably the best known natural colourant. It strengthens the hair as it coats the hair shaft.

If you have only a few white strands, henna can be used very effectively to conceal them.

Coffee or *Kathatha* (catechus) added to the henna paste gives hair a rich brown colour instead of a reddish tinge.

Chemical dyes have a toxic base and have been known to cause irritations and allergies. Before you dye your hair with chemical dyes, it is better to consult a specialist who could do the patch test and measure your sensitivity to the chemical.

Split Ends

When the cuticle breaks and dislodges at the end of the hair, the result is split ends.

Causes

Constant rubbing of the ends of the hair damages them and they split. This can happen due to any reason, for example, when you leave your hair open, two strands of hair rub against each other producing friction, thus causing split ends.

Visit a beautician to get your split ends trimmed.

A balanced, nutritious diet goes a long way in preventing split ends.

Lack of proper hair care and an imperfect diet can also lead to boils, sores, and lesions in the scalp. Ringworm or other fungal infections can also attack hair which is generally neglected. In all these cases, you must consult a doctor.

Hair, after all, is the crowning glory of one's personality. The scalp, on which healthy hair depends, is a sensitive, living tissue. It needs care and protection. All problems related to the scalp and hair, must be given immediate attention.

Pediculosis – Lice Infestation

Any slackness in cleanliness breeds lice infestation. A louse is a parasitic insect with six claw-like feet. It is grey in colour but turns brownish after sucking blood, which it does with two small trunk-like whiskers. A louse egg hatches in nine days and within a fortnight, the young ones attain maturity. Long hair is more prone to lice infestation. The back of the head itches when infested with lice, and itching causes abrasion of the scalp. Lice can be controlled by removing their eggs in the initial stages. Avoid using towels, soaps or combs of a person who has lice.

Nits (lice on the scalp) cause havoc in schools where lice infestation is common. The adult lice runs from one scalp to another, sticking eggs on the hair with a strong cement-like substance. The pearly nits look like sticky dandruff, but cannot be shaken off. Running a nail along the hair will not detach the eggs. The scalp infestation by lice induces scratching which in turn may cause bacterial infection. The insect lays eggs which are contained in a whitish ovoid receptacle called the nit, which is attached to the hair by a collar-like projection. The nit can be slid along the hair but not pulled off. The search for lice or nits in suspected cases of pediculosis of the scalp should be made on the back and sides of the head.

The lice can be killed with a single application of 1 per cent gamma-benzene hexachloride, or 2 per cent DDT emulsion or 25 per cent benzyl benzoate emulsion. The scalp should be washed after 24 hours, and the nits should be carefully removed with a comb as the ova are unaffected by these agents. The treatment may have to be repeated after a week or ten days. You may consult a doctor also.

A few ways for controlling lice are listed below:

- An anti-lice oil can be mixed with coconut (or mustard) oil and 0.2 per cent lindance (BHC) or 0.1 per cent pyrethrum essence. This oil can be rubbed well into the scalp to kill lice (ingredients can be purchased from a chemist).

- Mix talcum powder with 0.2 per cent pyrethrum dust in it (or add 10 per cent DDT). Sprinkle this powder on the hair before going to bed and rub it vigorously so that it reaches the roots. Cover your mouth, nose and eyes to protect them from the powder.
- Anti-louse lotion, either gammabenzene hexacholoride lotion or cream (Lorexane, Gammaexane) or malathion (Preioderma) will kill the eggs which can be removed by a comb with very fine teeth. One treatment is enough, but the

entire family should be treated and the hair examined regularly for a while. You may consult a doctor for the treatment.

The above-mentioned concoctions should be used at night. Tie a cloth around your head after applying any one of the medicines and let it remain at least for 24 hours. Before washing off, do not use soap or shampoo. Repeat this for a week and the lice and their eggs will be eliminated. Pediculosis pubis refers to infestation by a crab-shaped louse. In addition to the pubic area, it also affects the armpits, legs, a hairy chest, eyebrows and the eyelashes. Consult a doctor for the treatment of this infestation.

Tips for Hair Care

To ensure that your hair is clean and healthy, follow this simple 3-step formula regularly.

Step 1 - Cleansing

- Regular cleansing of your hair helps wash away the excess oil from your hair and scalp and removes the dead skin as well.
- Proper cleansing encourages healthy hair growth.
- Use a good shampoo and make sure you wash your hair at least once a week.

Step 2 - Toning

- To keep your body healthy, you need to exercise regularly. Similarly, your hair needs regular exercise too. Toning helps you do that.
- Toning of scalp and hair is achieved by gently massaging the head with your fingers, which helps in stimulating and invigorating the blood circulation required for the healthy growth of hair.

- Use a coconut, gooseberry *(amla)*, or olive- based hair oil, to gently massage your hair.

Step 3 - Conditioning

- The most important part of hair-care is conditioning – it is a restorative routine.
- If the hair is excessively stripped of moisture or oil due to harsh cleansing, exposure to the sun or application of harsh chemicals such as perm lotions, etc., the conditioning routine helps to restore and correct the imbalance. The kind of

conditioning required depends entirely on the physical condition of the hair.

- Another important aspect of effective care is the use of proper hair-care products.
- Different types of hair need different hair-care products. The use of wrong products is detrimental to the hair.
- Always use products made by reputed companies.
- Check on the date of manufacturing. Do not buy products more than a year old.

Ten Survival Steps for Great and Healthy Hair

- Wash your hair regularly and keep it clean.
- Massage your scalp regularly to ensure proper toning of the hair.
- Condition your hair with a good quality conditioner.
- Do not blow dry your hair very often. Let it dry naturally.
- Do not expose your hair to the sun or strong winds for a long time. Use a cap or umbrella to cover your hair if you are going to be in the open for a long time.

- Wash your hair with a mild shampoo and conditioner, if you have been swimming.
- Keep your hair in good shape and condition.
- Have a regular hair cut. It helps remove the broken ends and ensures even growth.
- Use a good quality hair colour and special hair rejuvenators.
- Tension and stress can cause hair fall.Learn to relax.
- Your emotions and feelings affect the health of your hair. Try to relax and be cheerful and watch your hair become beautiful.

- Yoga is also helpful.
- Follow a diet which is rich in vitamins A, E and B.

More Tips for Hair Care

Finger Combing

Comb your hair with your fingers to remove snarls and tangles before using the hair brush.

Proper Brushing of Hair

Bend forward, allowing the hair to fall in front of the face. Using only a wooden base natural bristle brush, bring the hair from the nape of the neck over the head and down to the ends. Then, stand straight again with the hair falling normally, and brush from the underside of the hairline down the strands to the ends. Now, brush the top layers into place with long, even strokes.

After each stroke, smooth the hair with your hands to reduce the static energy produced. Increase the number of strokes weekly, starting with five and increasing by one every week until you find a comfortable routine. If oiliness develops, reduce the number of strokes. Hair is weakest when it is wet and brushing can easily damage it; hence, brush your hair only when it has completely dried. Even when the hair is dry, always comb before brushing.

Combing

Separate the hair into small sections. With a wide-toothed comb, carefully work from the ends in a downward direction only. Use a wooden or a tortoise shell comb. Do not pull or yank the hair.

Drying

Dry your hair naturally. Avoid using hair dryers, as they spoil the texture of the hair.

Curling

Use regular hair rollers, winding hair loosely around them. Avoid electric rollers, hot combs, and curling irons, or use these on a cool setting. Pin curls or barrel curls are the safest and fastest methods of drying hair.

Shampooing

If your hair is dry and brittle, wet your hair, then coat with a light conditioner before shampooing. This acts as a buffer and helps protect the hair strand. Then shampoo, removing the dirt by gentle washing. Shampoos which are specially formulated with natural botanicals, and designed to clean the hair without stripping away its natural oils, are recommended.

Massage your head to increase the blood supply to the scalp and roots. Shampoo the hair regularly to remove unwanted residues of styling products and dirt from the environment.

Environment

Before going out to the beach or the pool, use a conditioner. This helps to protect the hair from the sun, chlorine and salt water. Wear a hat, cap or scarf if you can to protect the hair from over-exposure to the sun, salt or chlorinated water, wind or air pollution.

Trimming

Have your hair trimmed on a regular basis (approximately every two months). Trimming your hair regularly reduces the split ends.

Conditioning

Conditioning too often can cause the cuticle layer of the hair to lift, making the hair brittle and leading to breakage. Rather than conditioning every day, try a good conditioner once a week.

Styling

Your hair-style is a reflection of your personality and a wonderful way to express your individuality. Very often, conventional styling products contain alcohol or other harsh chemicals. These ingredients are used to keep the hair in place and to give the appearance of shiny healthy hair.

In the case of these chemical-based, mass-marketed products, the look achieved is only surface deep and they tend to damage the hair. There are highly specialized styling products which not only make your hair look great, but also impart essential minerals and vitamins to each strand, conditioning the hair as they hold it in place. They give it an incredible shine and bounce as well.

Sleeping

Even the way you sleep can affect your hair. Restless sleepers may actually be breaking their hair as they sleep.

If you are a restless sleeper, try a satin pillowcase so that the hair glides when you move in your sleep. On regular cotton cases, the hair can get caught and might even break.

Tying your hair up before going to sleep is also helpful. Hair should be put in a ponytail on top of the head. Always use rubber bands that are wrapped in cloth, commonly known as "scrunchies".

Tips for Long Hair

Hair grows in accordance with your body's chemistry, balance and well-being. It is a conception that after a certain point, the hair growth slows down. Patience and proper maintenance is the key, when you are planning to grow your hair long. It is very important to trim split ends. Also, use the right shampoos, conditioners and styling products in order to prevent split ends. Eat a well-balanced diet, work out, and supplement your diet with vitamins essential for healthy hair. Remember that hair is a natural fibre and is a natural reflection of your health and well-being. So if you are careless about your body, your hair will lack the look you desire. Treat your body with care, follow a proper hair care programme and supplement your diet with vitamins. You will soon see that with a little amount of patience and care, your hair will begin to look and feel great.

The number one problem affecting long hair is breakage, usually seen as shorter, fly-away strands, or split ends. From the moment you wake up, to the time you go to sleep and even as you sleep, there are many factors that can lead to hair breakage. One of the most common causes is poor maintenance—things like improper brushing and washing and infrequent trimming. Life-style factors, such as poor nutrition, stress, and even restless sleeping can also lead to hair damage.

The problem is that what many people think is good for their hair may actually be hurting it. Through proper care, using simple techniques and the right maintenance products, anyone can have long, beautiful, healthy locks.

HERBAL REMEDIES

For Manageable Hair

Ingredients

½ mashed avocado

1 tbs mayonnaise

- Mix together and apply to washed hair. Rinse thoroughly.

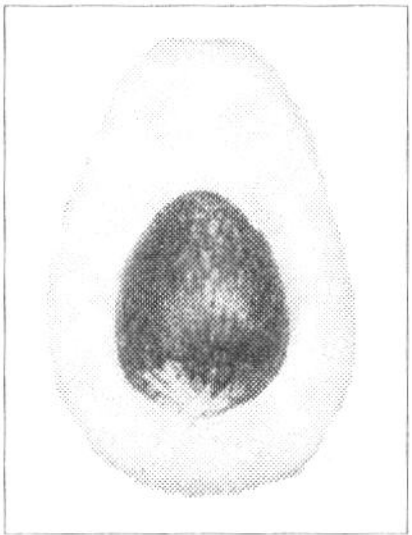

Avocado

For Healthy Hair

Solution I

Ingredients

100 g of *reetha* seeds
100 g of dried *amla* powder
100 g of dried *shikakai* powder
20 g of aloe vera juice
3 glasses of hot water

- Soak the *reetha* seeds in warm water and squeeze out the juice. Add the rest of the ingredients and use as a regular shampoo.

Solution II

- Mix 1 cup skimmed milk and an egg. Rub this mixture on your scalp. Rinse after five minutes.

Solution III

- Mix castor oil, glycerine and cider vinegar in a mild shampoo. Leave for twenty minutes.

Solution IV

- Mix cocunut oil or castor oil with lavender essence oil. Heat it till lukewarm. Apply on your hair and leave overnight. Shampoo the next day.

For Non-greasy Hair

Solution I

Ingredients

1/4 cup lemon juice

1/3 cup of your regular shampoo

- Mix together and shampoo as usual.

Solution II

- Take 2 tbs gram flour and 1 teaspoon of *shikakai* and mix with a cupful of coconut milk. Apply on your hair and scalp. Rinse after five minutes.

For Limp Hair

Solution I

- After washing your hair, massage with beer, concentrating on your scalp only.
- Do not rinse — this will give more volume to your hair.

Solution II

- Grind a few onions and some cabbage together and soak it overnight. Add

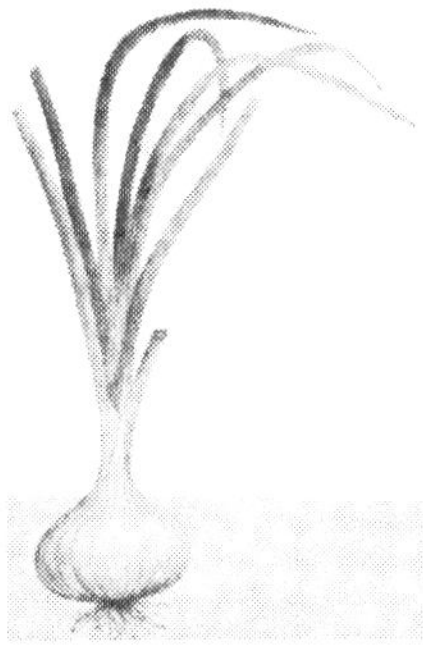

Onion

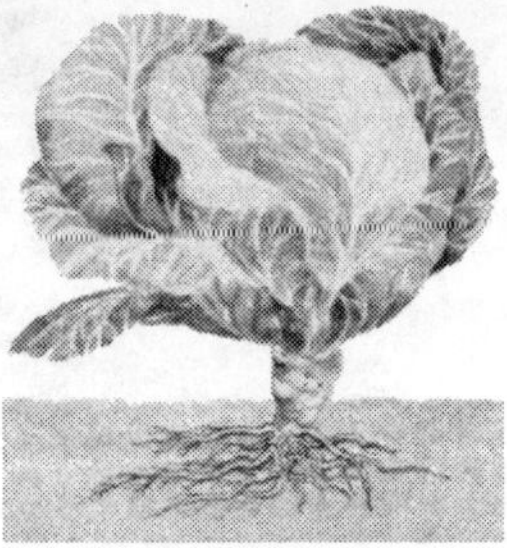

Cabbage

eau de cologne, *amla* or *Brahmi* oil to the paste. Apply and rinse after half an hour.

For Soft and Silky Hair

- Boil water with some tea leaves.
- Shower with this water, it will make your hair soft as silk.

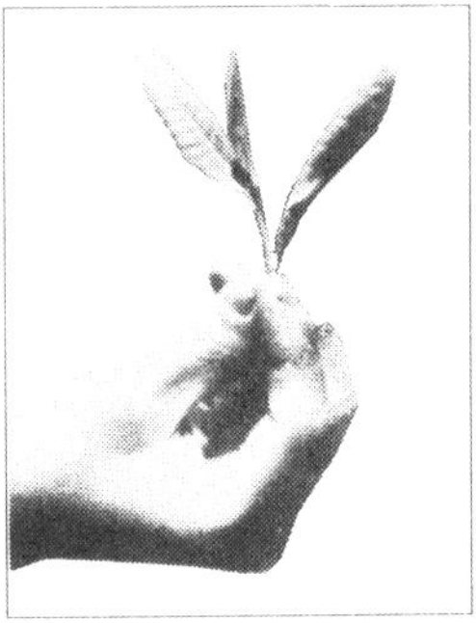

Tea Leaves

For Thick and Shiny Hair

Solution I

- Grind Hibiscus petals.
- Add the egg white of two eggs.
- Mix and apply to the hair and leave it on for half an hour.
- Shampoo as usual.

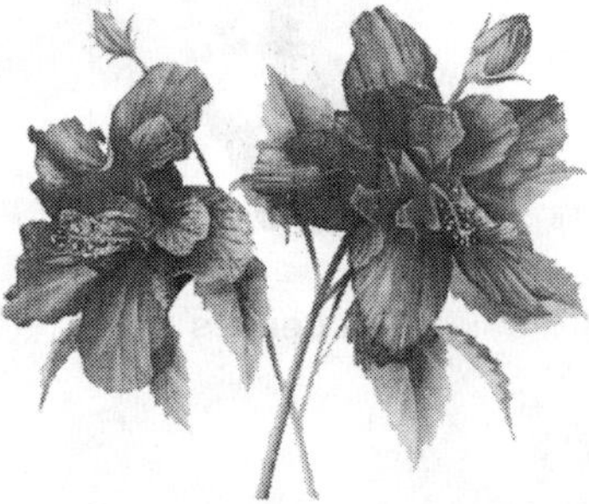

Hibiscus

Solution II

- Apply yoghurt on your hair and scalp.
- Shampoo after half an hour.

Solution III

- Mix a little mayonnaise in some hair oil.
- Massage your scalp with it and leave it on for half an hour.
- Wash your hair using a mild shampoo.

For Strengthening Hair Follicles

- Mix rosemary, thyme and water in the proportion of 1:1:10.

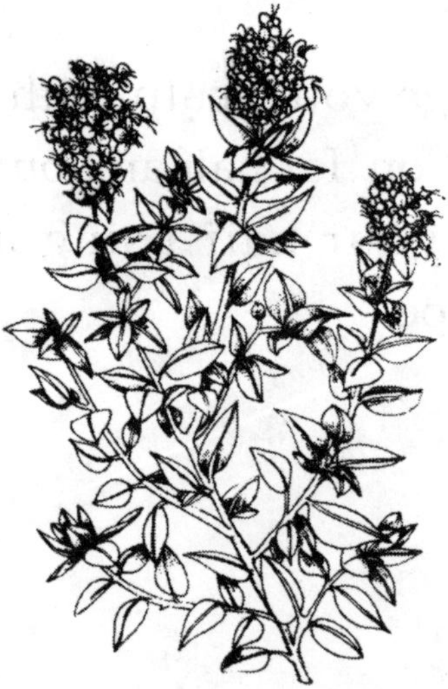

Thyme

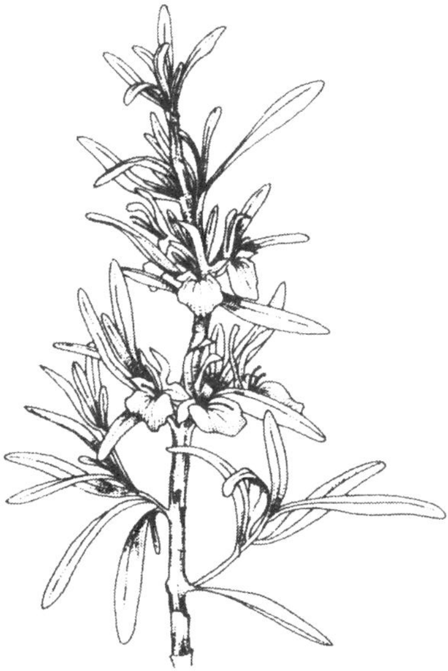

Rosemary

- Apply this on your scalp twice a day. Leave it on for an hour before rinsing with water.

For Preventing Hair Loss

Solution I

- Massage beetroot juice on your scalp. Do this regularly, every night.

Solution II

- Boil a few curry leaves in 100 ml of coconut oil.
- Use this decoction to massage your scalp and hair.
- Leave for an hour and shampoo as usual.
- For excellent results, try this twice a week.

Solution III

- Grind the peels of lemon, orange and pomegranate.
- Dry in the sun and mix the paste in coconut oil.
- Massage your scalp with this mixture.
- Leave it on for an hour before washing your hair.
- Using it twice a week, for six months will help in arresting falling hair.

Solution IV

- Rosemary oil can be used to massage the scalp, but avoid this remedy if you have oily hair.

Solution V

- Grind *amla* and make a paste with lemon juice.
- Rub this mixture on the scalp and leave it on for ten minutes.
- Shampoo as usual.
- Not only does this check hair fall, it also makes your hair long and dark.

For Thick and Black Hair

Solution I

Castor Oil Remedy

- Massage your hair and scalp with castor oil.
- Steam your head.
- Shampoo after half an hour.

Solution II

Vodka Remedy

Ingredients

1/3 cup vodka

1/3 cup of your favourite shampoo

- Mix together and shampoo as usual.

For a Clean Scalp

- Massage the scalp with undiluted apple cider vinegar.
- Leave it on for fifteen minutes before washing your hair.

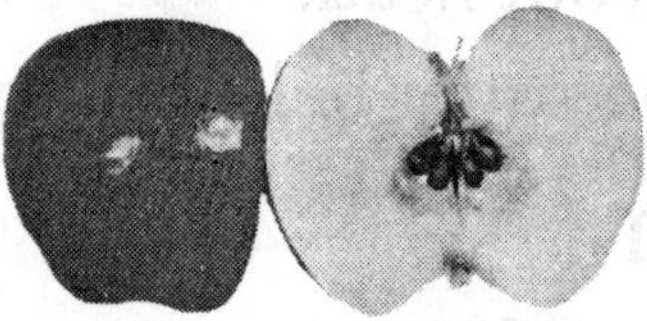

Apple

- It makes the hair and scalp absolutely clean.
- Do not try this more than once a week as this causes dryness.

For Thick Hair

Coconut Remedy

- Grind some coconut and squeeze the milk from the ground coconut.

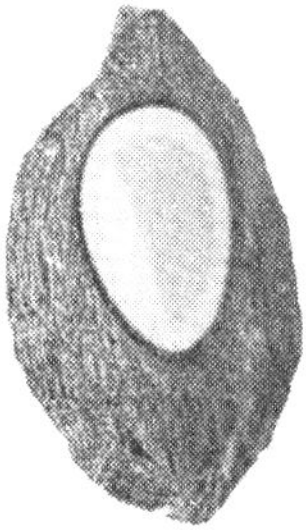

Coconut

- Boil the milk so that the water evaporates, leaving behind oil.
- Massage this oil on your scalp.
- Shampoo after an hour.

For Black Hair

Lemon - Tea Remedy

- Add lemon juice to boiled and strained tea-water.
- Use this as the final rinse.

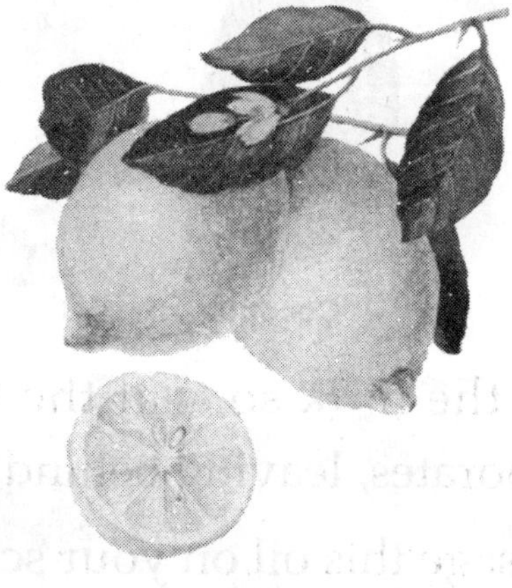

Lemon

For Glossy Hair

Solution I

- Boil 3/4 cup of beer till it becomes 1/4
- Cool it and add to your shampoo. Use as usual.

Solution II

- Extract celery juice.
- Apply evenly on the scalp.
- Rinse with water and use a mild shampoo.
- This also helps in increasing the length of your hair.

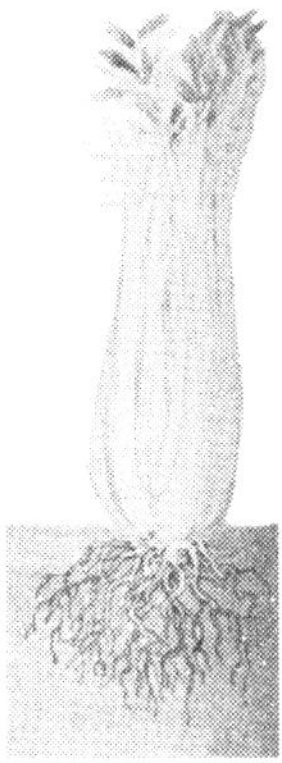

Celery

For Accelerating Hair Growth

- Make a thick paste of henna, yoghurt, eggs and lemon juice.
- Apply evenly all over your hair and scalp.
- Shampoo after an hour.
- This also helps in treating cases of hair loss.

For Adding Bounce to your Hair

- Soak 1 tbs of fenugreek seeds (*methi*) in water overnight.
- Grind this to a paste and rub on to your scalp.
- Shampoo after half an hour.
- After the shampoo, rinse your hair with a mixture of vinegar or lemon juice and water.

For Getting Rid of Split Ends

Solution I

Olive Oil Remedy

- Coat the ends of your hair with olive oil (about 1/3 of the way up) before going to bed.

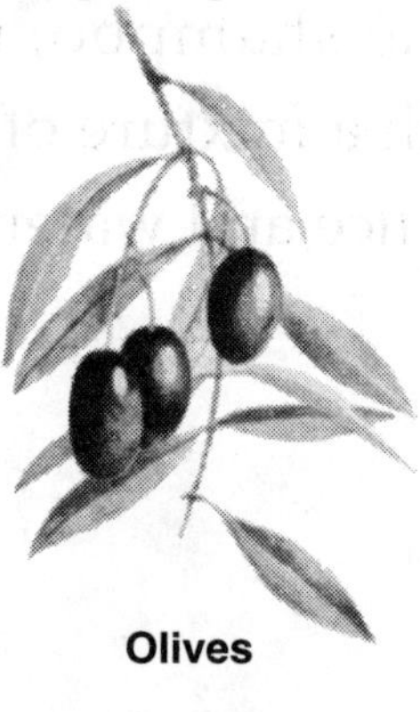

Olives

- Wash your hair the next morning, using a vitamin shampoo.
- Repeat this treatment two to three times in a week.

Solution II

Multiple Oil Remedy

- Mix castor oil, mustard oil and olive oil.
- Heat to make it lukewarm.
- Massage on the scalp and leave it on for half an hour.
- Steam with a hot towel and leave the oil on the hair for two hours.
- Shampoo as usual.

- Shampoo as usual.
- This also makes your hair soft and silky.

Solution III

Almond Oil Remedy

- Mix 1 tablespoon of almond oil, 1 teaspoon of honey and the yolk of an egg.

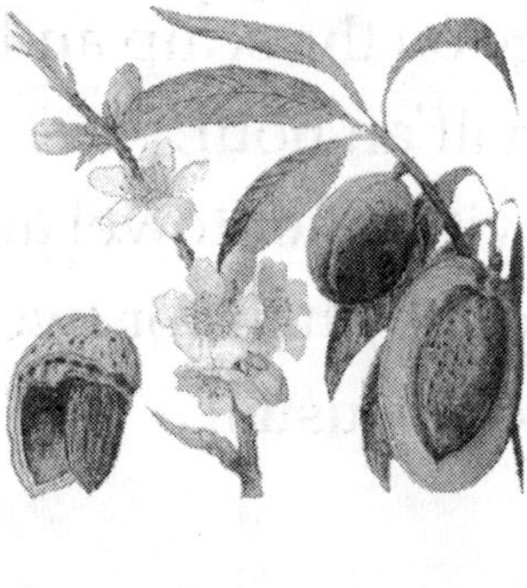

Almonds

- Shampoo your hair after an hour.

Tips

- Trim frequently.
- Avoid vigorous combing.

For Stiff Hair

- Use any conditioner that suits you, once a week.
- While drying your hair, give priority to the ends.
- Massage with warm coconut oil once a week before shampooing your hair.

For Getting Rid of Dandruff

Never wash your hair with boiling hot water. The extra heat on the scalp encourages dandruff formation.

Solution I

Carrot Juice Remedy

- Massage the scalp with carrot juice, once a week, before washing your hair.

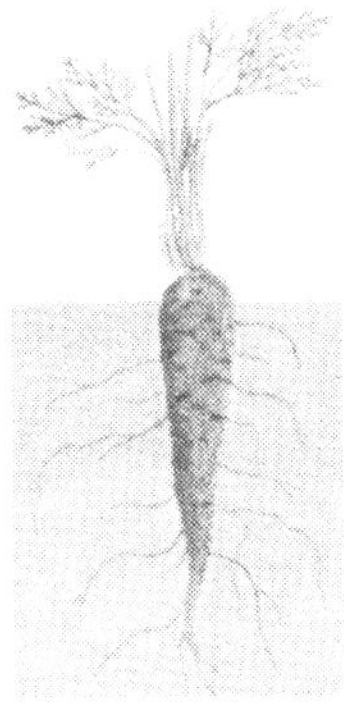

Carrot

Solution II

Eucalyptus and Clove Oil Remedy

- Eucalyptus and clove oil mixed in the proportion of 3:1 should be massaged into the scalp every night.

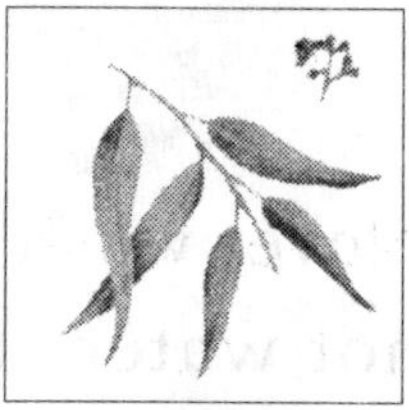

Eucalyptus leaves

Solution III

Rose Water Remedy

- For oily dandruff, mix rose water and eau de cologne in equal parts and massage your scalp with it. Leave it on for an hour before shampooing.

Solution IV

Sour Curd Remedy

- Apply sour curd on the scalp and leave it on for half an hour. Then shampoo your hair.

Solution V

Warm Coconut Oil Remedy

- Apply warm coconut oil to your hair and leave it overnight. Mix salt in a little lemon juice and apply on your scalp. Wash it off after an hour.

Solution VI

Gram flour (Besan) Pack

- Mix two tablespoons of gram flour (*besan*), sour curd and an egg white. Apply evenly and then wash after twenty minutes. Try this treatment for six months, once every week, and you will see the difference.

Solution VII

Lemon Juice Remedy

- Mix 3 tablespoons of lemon juice with 1/4 cup of coconut oil and massage the scalp with it. Shampoo after an hour.

Solution VIII

Mouthwash Pack

- Mix one part of mouthwash (that is labelled antiseptic) with nine parts of water and massage it on the scalp. Rinse after ten minutes.

Solution IX

Trifala Pack

- Mix 1 teaspoon of *trifala* in a glass of water and boil for three minutes. Mix an equal amount of cider vinegar to this decoction. Massage with it and leave it on for the night. Wash with a mild shampoo.

Solution X

Fenugreek (Methi) Pack

- Soak 100 g of fenugreek seeds (*methi*) overnight. In the morning make a paste and use this paste as a shampoo.

Solution XI

Beetroot Juice Remedy

- Apply beetroot juice to your scalp and leave it on for an hour before washing your hair.

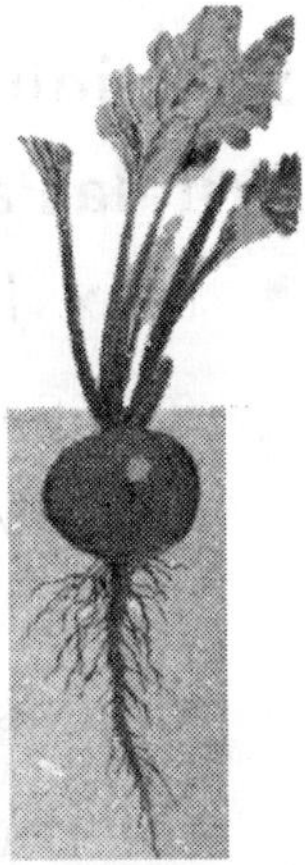

Beetroot

Solution XII

Gram flour (Besan) - Honey Pack

- Add a few drops of honey to some *besan* and make it into a paste with vinegar. Apply and rinse and shampoo after five minutes.

Solution XIII

Henna - Shikakai Pack

- Take a few henna leaves, some *amla, shikakai, baherha* and boil them together. Mash the pulp and apply to the roots. Leave it on for half an hour and then shampoo your hair.

For Oily Hair

- Mix five tablespoons of henna with two tablespoons of yogurt and a little bit of sugar.
- Make it into a thick paste – add a little water if required.
- Apply evenly on the scalp and hair and leave it on for half an hour.
- Wash, using a mild shampoo.

For Dry Hair

Solution I

Henna Remedy

- Make a paste of eight table-spoons of henna, one tablespoon of oil and the appropriate quantity of lukewarm milk.
- Apply evenly and leave it on for fifteen minutes. Then shampoo as usual.

Solution II

Oil Remedy

- Massage coconut or olive oil and steam your hair.
- Massage once again and shampoo as usual.

Solution III

Milk Remedy

- If allergic to oil, you could massage your hair and scalp with milk and then shampoo after an hour.

Tips

- Avoid using a hair dryer.
- Allow the hair to dry naturally.
- Use soft combs.

- Use a conditioner once in two weeks.
- Take a high protein diet.

For Revitalising Hair

- Massage the contents of some vitamin E capsules on the scalp.
- Leave it on for half an hour.
- Rinse thoroughly with lukewarm water.

For Preventing Summer Rashes on the Scalp

- Mix castor oil, seasame oil and coconut oil in equal proportions.
- Apply evenly on the scalp and leave it on for a while.
- Rinse with cold water.

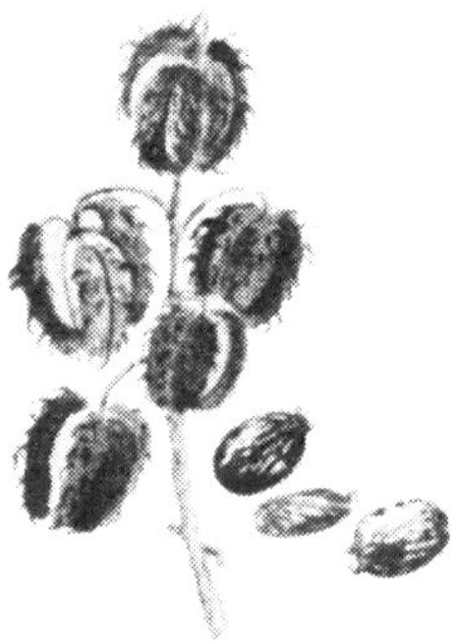

Castor Beans

Herbal Hair Care Solutions for Grey Hair

Henna is a natural dye. Henna applications, while colouring the hair, also add beauty and bounce to it, leaving it supple, shiny and easy to manage. It is also a very effective cleanser both for the hair and the scalp, which is an essential pre-requisite for healthy hair.

Henna — For colouring Grey Hair

- Make a paste of equal quantities of henna and tea, one egg, one tablespoon of castor oil, a tablespoon of *amla* powder and one teaspoon of coffee powder.

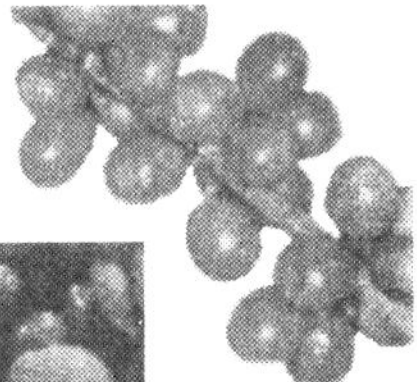

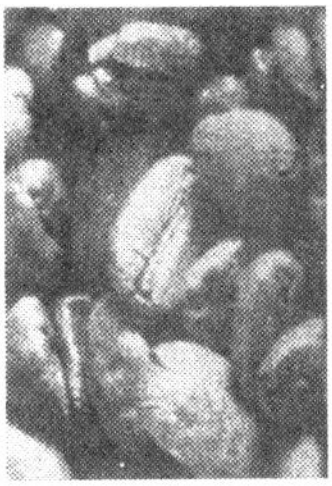

Coffee

- Apply evenly all over the scalp and hair and leave it on for a few hours.
- Rinse with cold water and then shampoo.

Oil For Grey Hair

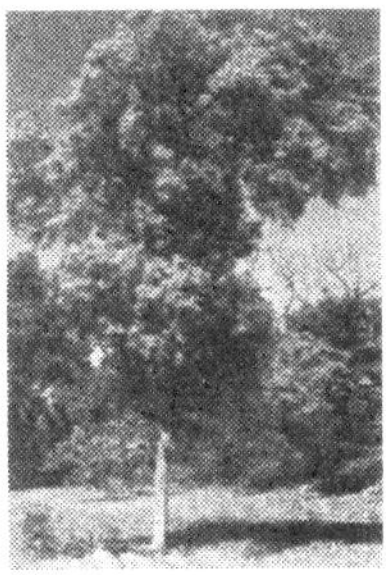

Sandalwood Tree

- Mix 100g of castor oil with 1 ounce of sandalwood powder and 1 ounce of coffee powder, and heat for twenty minutes. Cool and strain. Apply regularly on your scalp and hair. It prevents greying of hair.

For a Darker Shade

- Add a little amount of walnut paste to the henna mixture that you use for dyeing your hair.

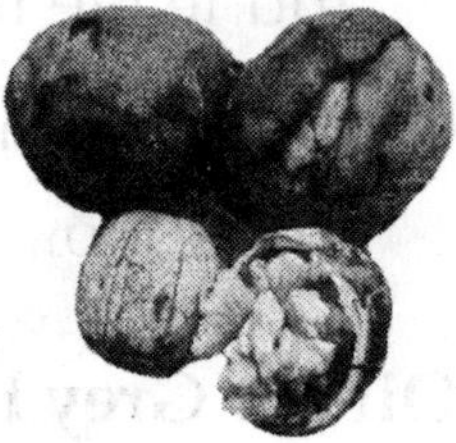

Walnut

- This would give a darker shade to your hair

For a Tinge of Copper

- Mix a few drops of eucalyptus oil to the henna paste and leave it for five minutes.
- Apply the paste evenly all over the scalp and hair.
- This would give a nice tinge of copper to your hair.

AYURVEDIC REMEDIES

Solutions from Ayurveda

In India, the references to the curative properties of some herbs in the *Rig Veda* seem to be the earliest record of the use of plants in medicine.

Feuerbach teaches us the basic principle of Ayurveda:

> *In the perishable petals of the flower there resides more spirit and life than in the lumpish granite boulder that has defied the wear and tear of thousand years.*

Here are a few ayurvedic remedies for dandruff and greying hair.

For Dandruff

An oil prepared from *Dhattura* leaves or seeds should be applied on the scalp, as a cure for dandruff. *Dhattura* leaves or seeds are available in the market in the name of *Durdur Patradi Taila (Arya Vaidya Shala, Kottakal)*.

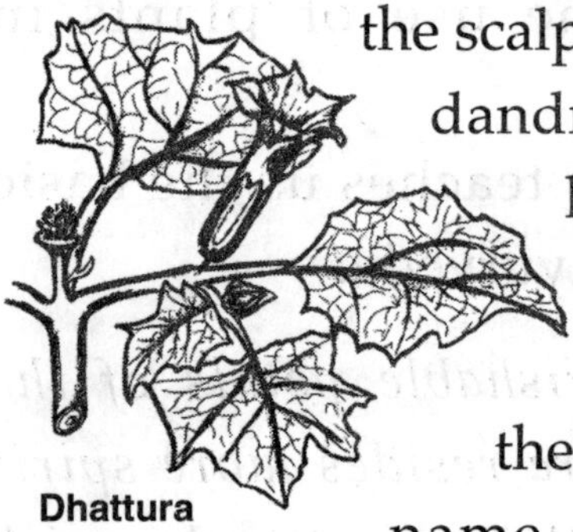

Dhattura

Warning — It is a dangerous drug if taken internally. It should be kept away from children.

For Greying Hair

Bhringaraja (Eclipta alba) and *Amalaki* (Emblica officinalis) should be taken in a powder form in a dose of one teaspoon each, twice daily, with milk or ghee. He/she is advised to take plenty of milk. The patient should avoid pungent and sour things like curds and spicy food. Prepared medicines like *Nasrasimha Rasayana* can be administered in a dose of one teaspoonful daily with milk.

The juice obtained from the leaves of *Bilva* (Aeglemarwelos corr) can also be applied externally. An application of the leaves of white *gunja* with *Bhringaraja* (Eclipta alba) will produce the same effect.

Hot water should never be used for washing hair. The water should either be lukewarm or cold. The patient must avoid anxiety, hurry, worry and excitement. If he/she suffers from a chronic cold and sinusitis, then these must be treated properly.

Treat your hair well and it will be your crowning glory. A little neglect can mean falling or greying hair, dandruff, split ends, dull and lack-lustre hair.

YOGIC REMEDIES

Yoga and Hair Care

The following asanas work wonders for the hair.

Kukkuta Asana

The Sanskrit word 'kukkuta' means a cock in English, and hence the name Kukkuta asana for the posture, which reminds one of a cock.

Method

Sit in the posture of Padmasana – sit on the ground with your legs stretched forward and your back

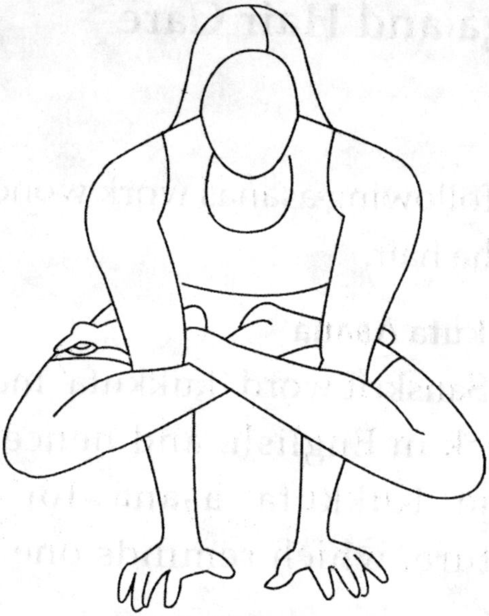

Kukkuta Asana

straight. Put the left foot on the right thigh and the right foot on the left thigh, so that the heels of the feet touch the abdomen.

Put your hands through the gap between the calves and the thighs, and place the palms of your hands on the floor. Now try to balance the weight of your body on your palms and do this for a minute at least.

Shuturmurgha Asana

This asana is also very effective for the instant growth of hair.

Warning

Pregnant ladies should not try this, though after the delivery of the baby, they can try it to keep their body and hair fit and healthy.

Method

Stand straight and then bend from the waist. Try to touch the floor with your fingers, making sure that your back is straight. You can achieve this posture with a little practice.

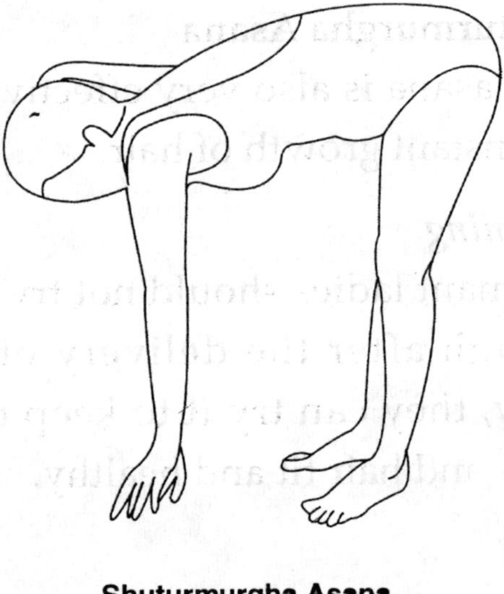

Shuturmurgha Asana

If you have long hair, then let it loose and allow it to fall on to the floor. Do this for a few seconds and then resume your standing posture.

Vajrasana

Vajra means thunderbolt and this asana makes the body very strong and healthy.

Method

Sit on your heels, with the knees, ankles and toes touching the floor. Place the palms on your knees and keep your back straight. Slowly take a deep breath and relax, expanding your chest and tightening the

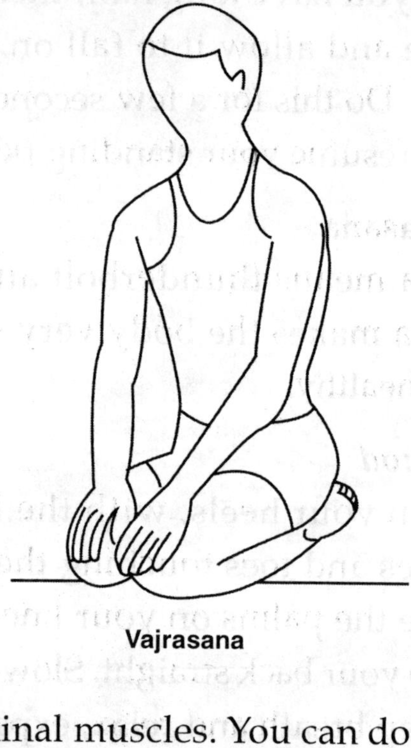

Vajrasana

abdominal muscles. You can do this asana even after taking your meals.

Chakrasana

Chakra means a wheel and since the posture of chakrasana looks like a wheel, the name of this asana is chakrasana.

Method

Lie on your back with your legs straight. Bend the legs so that the heels are near your buttocks. Bend your arms backwards so that the palms touch the floor with the fingers pointing towards the shoulder. Take a deep breath and raise your head and trunk off the floor, arching your body so that

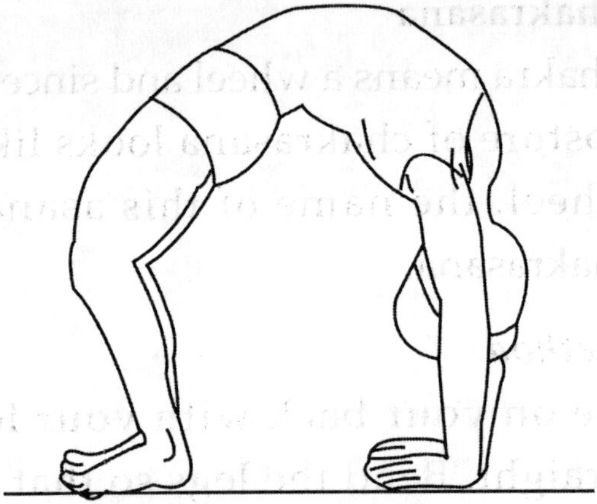

Chakrasana

your back is off the floor and your body weight is balanced on your palms and feet.

Do not overstretch your back for your may strain it. Stay in the final pose for as long as it is comfortable.

Conclusion

This is a complete book on Hair Care for anyone and everyone who wants healthy hair. All kinds of Herbal, Ayurvedic and Yogic remedies are described in detail – how to make the mask, how to apply it, and for how long, etc.

How well you look after your hair – whether you follow the precribed remedy as described – depends on you. Hence the health of your hair ultimately rests with you. The choice is yours, and with a little regular care you can have what you want.

OTHER TITLES IN THE SERIES

All You Wanted to Know About

Gems

Graphology

Numerology

Palmistry

Astrology

Vaastushastra

Feng Shui

Hypnosis

Dowsing

Increasing Memory Power

The Prophecies of Nostradamus

[illegible]THROUGH

Pastor Francis

James Osborn Nanjo

You are very special

[illegible]

18-09-03

EMMANUEL HOUSE
London, United Kingdom

Breakthrough Prayers

Published by
Emmanuel House
PO Box 15022
London
SE5 7ZL

All scriptures, unless otherwise stated, are taken from the *King James Version* of the Bible.

ISBN 1 900529 08 4

Cover design by Efih
Printed in England by Cox & Wyman Ltd., Reading, Berkshire

CONTENTS

ACKNOWLEDGEMENTS

Over the years, my life and ministry have been shaped and influenced by many people and in diverse ways through love, encouragement, wise counsel and support. I thank God for you all.

I am very grateful to Rev. Sammy Amponsah of *Restored Pentecostal Ministry* (Ghana) for encouraging me to start writing. I also thank God for the special help I have received in diverse ways from Rev. & Mrs. Ntorikansah and the *Living Flames Baptist Church* (London).

Bishop & Rev. (Mrs.) Duncan Williams of *Action Faith Chapel* (Ghana), your heart of love and commitment towards my life in many ways have really blessed me. Rev. & Mrs. Ampiah Kwofi and the family of *Global Revival Church* (Ghana), I am proud to be a part of you. I am very thankful to God for Rev. & Mrs. Kofi Banful of *Praise Chapel* (London) for their kindness. I thank God also for Mr. & Mrs. Sarpon (London), friends of *Omega Revolution Generation* and *World Restoration Ministries*.

I am grateful to God for the input of

Rev. Tokunbo Emmanuel of *Emmanuel House* in the production of this book and for Rev. Bernard Ankomah of *World Rescue Ministries* (USA) for kindly writing the foreword. I am privileged to have contacts with you all and many others I have not mentioned. God bless you all.

Finally and most importantly, I am grateful to God for granting me this opportunity to express his grace upon my life. Lord Jesus, I am thankful to you. Holy Spirit, thank you for inspiring me to put this material together. To God be all the glory for the great things He has done!

* * * * *

DEDICATION

With my heart filled with gratitude and appreciation beyond my ability to express in words, I gratefully dedicate this book to the founder and leader of Global Revival Ministries and Ampiah Kwofi World Outreach, ***Rev. Robert Ampiah Kwofi****, to whom I was super-naturally directed to submit to as a son in the Lord. The spirit of prayer was transferred to me the effect of which includes the production of this book, Breakthrough Prayers. To God be all the Honour. Thanks again Papa Robert.*

FOREWORD

The Word of God is the only reliable solution to the problems of our fast and changing world. There is no better gift of love Evangelist James Osborn could give us all at this challenging time of life than the simplified golden keys for total victory disclosed in *Breakthrough Prayers*.

Read this book. Believe its contents. Apply the principles it teaches and expect nothing less than a God-given breakthrough in your life.

- Bernard Ankomah
President, World Rescue Ministries
Atlanta, USA

PERSONAL WORD

I am on a divine mission in this generation, commissioned from heaven with solutions for suffering humanity. We serve a God who has the answers to people's many questions and prayers.

By the grace and direction of God, I have put this material together so that anyone who reads it may experience a lift from poverty to prosperity, barrenness to fruitfulness, shame to glory.

Your life will never remain the same as you practically put to work the Biblical principles in this book. You will find in it choice words in line with God's Word that can form part of your language of prayer.

You will surely experience a breakthrough in every dimension of your life, in Jesus' name, and your life will never remain the same again as you diligently engage your heart and mind in *Breakthrough Prayers*. May the Lord bless you richly.

James Osborn Nanjo
October, 1999

SECTION ONE:

DEVELOPING A BREAKTHROUGH MENTALITY

DOMINION OVER PROBLEMS

"WHEN THE ENEMY SHALL COME IN LIKE A FLOOD, THE SPIRIT OF THE LORD SHALL LIFT UP A STANDARD AGAINST HIM"

(ISAIAH 59:19)

Refuse to see problems overtake you. Connect your spirit to this word: *"When the devil comes like a flood, the Holy Ghost will raise a standard higher than the flood to rescue you"*. I encourage you to always visualize what God has already put in place for you rather than what the devil is trying to do.

Never be discouraged or frustrated by problems. Deny problems the ability to steal your joy and happiness. **Always see the Spirit of God lifting a banner of victory on your behalf.** Friend, press on in life, for I am very confident that you **cannot** and **will not** fail.

DOMINION OVER CURSES

"CHRIST HATH REDEEMED US FROMTHE CURSE OF THE LAW, BEING MADE A CURSE FOR US. FOR IT IS WRITTEN, CURSED IS EVERY ONE THAT HANGETH ON A TREE"

(GALATIANS 3:13)

Anyone under the curse of a particular problem has lost dominion over the circumstance. **God wants believers to live above curses.** It is not His will for any believer to remain perpetually under a curse.

We have received redemption from the curses listed in Deuteronomy 28:15-65. Your time has come to **boldly** declare your stand and come out from under that curse. Make this prayer confession as follows:

I AM NOT SUBJECT TO SICKNESS

I AM NOT SUBJECT TO BARRENNESS

I AM NOT SUBJECT TO IMPOTENCY

I AM NOT SUBJECT TO DEFEAT

It does not matter how serious your situation is now; if you will confess and believe in what God says about you, there will be a change for the better.

Be quickened in your spirit. Rise up in faith, never to believe in the devil's lie again. **Right now, I see doors open in your life; you are about to inherit every delayed miracle in your life, in Jesus' name.**

DOMINION OVER POVERTY

You are either rich or poor in this life depending on your application of the truths of God. You can prosper when you know what the word of God says about prosperity. When you believe the word and set your heart on it, you will experience dominion over poverty.

What does the Word say?

"BELIEVE IN THE LORD YOUR GOD, SO SHALL YE BE ESTABLISHED. BELIEVE HIS PROPHETS, SO SHALL YE PROSPER"

(2 CHRONICLES 20:20)

"AS LONG AS HE SOUGHT THE LORD, GOD MADE HIM TO PROSPER"

(2 CHRONICLES 26:5)

Poverty should not be your portion if you believe in *genuine* prophets of God. Again, you will prosper when you seek the Lord to a point where no one else can touch your heart like He does. These divine truths can empower you for prosperity.

Do not identify your self with poverty. Instead, see your self prospering in every area of your life.

Pray and confess: *I believe in the true prophets of God. I believe that they are agents of God for prosperity. Therefore, I cannot be poor. I choose to prosper. I will seek the face of God always. I believe that the Lord will prosper the work of my hands.*

DOMINION OVER SICKNESS

"WHO FORGIVETH ALL THINE INIQUITIES, WHO HEALETH ALL THY DISEASES"

(PSALM 103:3)

There are forces of wickedness released from hell to fight your health with varieties of diseases. You can gain power over any of these diseases if you understand that Jesus has forgiven us all our iniquities, and has made provision for our sound health.

If God has forgiven you all your iniquities, then He has likewise healed you of all your diseases. Please, don't question the Bible because this is the truth. Receive and operate it by faith.

Tell the devil that you cannot be sick because your sins have been forgiven. Tell him that you don't expect any sickness because Jesus has healed all your diseases.

Accept the fact that your sins have been washed away by the blood of Jesus and believe that as a result, you **cannot** and **will**

not be sick.

Moreover, this is what the Bible says:

"IF THOU WILT DILIGENTLY HEARKEN TO THE VOICE OF THE LORD THY GOD, AND WILT DO THAT WHICH IS RIGHT IN HIS SIGHT, AND WILT GIVE EAR TO HIS COMMANDMENTS, AND KEEP ALL HIS STATUTES, I WILL PUT NONE OF THESE DISEASES UPON THEE, WHICH I HAVE BROUGHT UPON THE EGYPTIANS: FOR I AM THE LORD THAT HEALETH THEE"

(EXODUS 15:26)

You can enjoy a sickness-free life and live in a sickness-free zone. The first part of the above Scripture clearly spells out what you must do for God to deliver you from sickness. Let's consider point by point what we must do.

IF YOU LISTEN CAREFULLY TO THE VOICE OF THE LORD.

IF YOU DO WHAT IS RIGHT IN HIS EYES.

IF YOU PAY ATTENTION TO HIS COMMANDS.

IF YOU KEEP ALL HIS DECREES.

When you fulfill these four requirements, God will not bring on you any of the diseases He brought on the Egyptians. We serve a God that heals the sicknesses of his people. When you come to Him and recognize Him as the Healer, He will surely heal you.

Now confess it boldly. **I do what is right in the sight of God. I pay attention to His commands and keep His decrees. Therefore, God will not put any of the Egyptian diseases upon me.** God loves me and I love him. I am healed from all my diseases today in Jesus' mighty name.

DOMINION OVER FEAR

Some people are under the oppression of the devil not because of any bad thing they have done, but because they entertain fear in their lives. Such people harbour the fear of insecurity, fear of the unknown, fear of the known, fear of the future, etc. There are many kinds of fear that the devil is using to oppress people today.

There is a massive operation of the activities of Satan against you than ever before. He will threaten you with problems so that you can surrender to fear. The moment you begin to fear, the devil will be free to gain access into your life. **No matter the problems you face, do not fear.**

"YEA, THOUGH I WALK THROUGH THE VALLEY OF THE SHADOW OF DEATH, I WILL FEAR NO EVIL"

(PSALM 23:4)

Fear not because Jesus is your shepherd and He cares for you. Boldly declare: *I will not fear sickness. I will not fear any form of problem.* Proclaim with confidence: ***Satan cannot make me fear in any area of my life!***

"THE LORD IS MY LIGHT AND MY SALVATION; WHOM SHALL I FEAR? THE LORD IS THE STRENGTH OF MY LIFE; OF WHOM SHALL I BE AFRAID?"

(PSALM 27:1)

Confess and believe that the Lord is your light of healing; He is your salvation. Confess that the Lord is the strength of your life and you will not fear anything.

I encourage you to take hold of whatever the Scriptures say about your life. Believe it without fear. In every situation of life, you need knowledge about what God has said. From the discovery of His Word, you can gain dominion over the enemy.

We must not be comfortable in the face of so many challenges in our world. Let's confront the enemy in prayer for God's will to be established. *I pray that you will be empowered from henceforth to exercise authority over fear of failure and death; that every new day in your life will enjoy the mercies of Jehovah.*

SECTION TWO:

DEVELOPING A PRAYER LIFE FOR BREAKTHROUGHS

POSITIVE CONFESSION

Positive confessions release positive things in the lives of believers. **Until you exercise authority over your needs and expectations through positive confession, you may never see your desires fulfilled.**

You must also be sure that your confession does not conflict with the Word of God, but that both of them are in agreement.

"THAT IF THOU SHALT CONFESS WITH THY MOUTH THE LORD JESUS, AND SHALT BELIEVE IN THINE HEARTH THAT GOD HATH RAISED HIM FROM THE DEAD, THOU SHALT BE SAVED"

(ROMANS 10:9)

Believing in the heart is the key for the activation of positive confession. You must first believe in your heart that God is able to do exceedingly, abundantly, beyond what you can ever dream or think about before you make any confession about it.

Salvation is the product of confession. The original interpretation for the word *salvation* means healing, deliverance, preserverance, well-doing and wholeness of spirit, soul and body. When you make positive confessions in line with God's Word, all these will be your portion.

Your mouth is an agent of miracles in your life through positive confession. Whatever the Bible says concerning your life, just believe and confess it and you will see it come to pass. As you make powerful Scriptural confessions for redemption in every area of your life, you will see the Holy Ghost at work with undeniable proofs of your miracle.

"ALSO I SAY UNTO YOU, WHOSOEVER SHALL CONFESS ME BEFORE MEN, HIM SHALL THE SON OF MAN ALSO CONFESS BEFORE THE ANGELS OF GOD"

(LUKE 12:8)

Jesus, referred to in the above Scripture as the Son of man, must confess you before the angels of God for protection and intervention against all the calculations and setups of the devil. However, this will not be done until you shamelessly declare your stand as a child of God.

If you cannot show through positive confession that you are proud to be connected to Jesus, you will never have the privilege of Him confessing you before God and the angelic host of heaven. Whenever Christ confesses you before the angels, they are discharged from heaven to speedily work on your behalf.

I pray that your angels will be discharged in time to quench all unquenchable fiery attacks of the devil - as you confess your faith in Jesus.

Friends, this is the secret of dominion - the power of positive confession. The devil may not fear every believer, but he fears those who know their goodly heritage and can boldly confess it among men.

It is about time that you confess the things you have been desiring for a long time. Do not give up confessing them until they come to pass. Believe and confess that your needs are met and you will surely receive what you confess.

"WHOSOEVER THEREFORE, SHALL CONFESS ME BEFORE MAN, HIM WILL I CONFESS ALSO BEFORE MY FATHER WHICH IS IN HEAVEN"

(MATTHEW 10:32)

This is a powerful tool for enthronement and dominion in Christ Jesus. It is a powerful secret we have to understand and apply for easy access into the promises of God.

In the first Scripture we considered, Jesus said that He will confess you before the angels of God - the supernatural, heavenly agents who ensure God's purposes in the natural realms. In other words, you must be recommended by Jesus to the angels before you can enjoy total angelic ministry.

This time, Jesus is saying that if you confess him publicly before men, He will confess you, not just to the angels, but to your Creator, God the Father.

If you learn to always make positive confessions with your mouth, Jesus will also give a witness about you to God for promotion, increase, expansion and so on.

There are a lot of things that the Father wants to do for you, but you need the Son to confess or talk about you as a reminder to the Father - even though the Father needs no remindal.

Anytime you confess that God provides for all your needs, Jesus will confess the same to the Father, and He (the Father) will respond by making abundant provisions available for you.

Your confession, therefore, is a controller of your destiny. If you want to see powerful things unfold in your life, then it is time that you confess all manner of good things into your life. Let's get started!

CONFESSION PRAYER

I pray and confess that I am more than a conqueror. I confess that I am undeniable, indestructible and unquenchable in God. I believe and confess that I shall not be barren in anyway; that I am prosperous and great. I know and confess that no weapon fashioned against me will prosper; that the Lord will lift a standard against anything that stands against my assignment on planet earth. I confess that in Christ, I am a great personality.

I believe and confess that I am anointed and the devil cannot touch my life. I confess that I will not lose focus and concentration in my calling. I know that I am too hot for the devil to handle.

You can join your faith with these prophetic declarations and pray the same prayers for your self concerning any area of your life, and you will see amazing wonders take place in your life in the name of Jesus, Amen.

PRAYER FOR ANOINTING

I believe and confess that I shall be anointed with fresh oil and my horn shall be exalted like the horn of a unicorn. I pray and confess that my head will never lack ointment and my garment will always be white. I believe that because I love righteousness and hate iniquity, I shall be anointed with the oil of joy above my fellows.

I confess that every yoke upon my life is destroyed because of the anointing. The yoke-destroying power of God demolishes every yoke over my family, my business and my marriage, in Jesus' mighty name, Amen.

PRAYER FOR LONG LIFE

I pray and confess that with long life will God satisfy me and show me the fulness of His saving power. I confess that as the number of my days on earth are, so shall my strength be with corresponding wisdom, grace, and abilities.

I will not die but live to declare the works of the Lord and His glory. God will not cast me away nor forsake me in my old age. He will still remember me when I am advanced in years. He will satisfy my mouth with good things and renew my youth as an eagle. I believe with all my heart that the Lord will keep all my bones and not one of them will be broken in Jesus' mighty name.

I believe that when I am old and grey-headed, God will not forsake me until I show his strength and power to the next generation. In Jesus' name, Amen.

PRAYER FOR PROTECTION

I believe and confess that I am divinely protected by God. I believe that the jealously of the Lord protects the unction upon my life and ministry.

The Lord shall deliver me from every trap and from every deadly calculation of the wicked one. I confess in the name of Jesus that the Lord shall cover me with His feathers, and under His wings will I trust for protection.

I trust and confess that he will give his angels charge over me and my family, to keep us in all our ways. They will keep us in their hands and none of us will strike our foot on invisible rocks.

I confess that because I have set my face upon the Lord, He will surely deliver me from every attack and programme of the enemy. With my eyes will I behold and see the reward of the wicked - none of them shall come upon my dwelling place.

I believe and confess that I am divinely

protected by the blood of Jesus. That my destiny is secured - my health, business, marriage and vision is heavily secured by the comprehensive insurance of the blood of Jesus.

I confess that I am covered by the efficacy of the blood of Jesus. My life and all the things that concern me are protected by the finger of God, in Jesus' mighty name, Amen.

PRAYER FOR ESTABLISHMENT

I pray and confess that wherever my feet shall step, the Lord shall give it to me as my inheritance. I pray for the increase and constant flow of wisdom and knowledge for my establishment in all areas of my life.

I confess that I am like a tree planted by the rivers of water. I will therefore produce good fruit in my season. I will never wither and whatever I do will prosper.

I confess that the God of Israel will establish me in an unlimited flow of the anointing. That I shall be established in my marriage, education, career, ministry, business and dreams.

I confess that I am established in righteousness and holiness, that I am established in the unlimited power of the Holy Ghost. I am perpetually established in the presence of the Lord and I shall not be moved by anything. Thank you Jesus for establishing all my ways by your word, in your holy name I pray, Amen.

PRAYER
FOR PROMOTION

I believe and confess that I have favour with God and favour with men and that promotion is due to me in every area of my life. I confess that I will be promoted at my workplace and in my walk with God.

Promotion comes not from the east, nor from the west, nor from the south, but God, the righteous Judge, brings one down and lifts up another. I confess that the time of my lifting is **now.** I will not be denied of my lift and raise into greatness. I pray and believe that I have been lifted from one perdestile unto another.

I confess that I have been highly exalted above all principalities and powers, and that I sit together with Christ Jesus in heavenly places. I confess that I have been promoted from one level of anointing to another. I confess that I am blessed and highly exalted by God for exploits in Jesus' precious name, Amen.

PRAYER FOR GREATNESS

I confess that the Lord has increased my greatness on every side and has comforted me in life. I pray and believe that the Lord will exalt my horn as the horn of the unicorn and grant me the strength of a mighty man of valour.

I confess that nothing in the world can humiliate my greatness, because greater is He that is in me than he that is in the world. I confess that as I remain a faithful servant of God, the Lord will make me great among men.

I trust and pray that the Lord, through me, shall build a great family, Church and nation. The Lord shall build a great people to his glory through my greatness. I am great because I serve a great God.

I believe and confess that I was recreated for greatness in the image of my Creator and I exercise my authority over anything that stands in my way of greatness, in the mighty name of Jesus, Amen.

PRAYER FOR RESTORATION

I confess and claim total restoration of every lost gifting and anointing upon my life. I confess and believe that I am totally restored from diseases into good health. I am restored from poverty into prosperity. I am restored from barrenness into fruitfulness. I am restored from prayerlessness into effective prayfulness. I confess that I have been totally restored from defeat of any kind into victories of every kind.

I confess and believe that I am restored from the bondage of sin into dominion over sin. I am restored from carnality into righteousness. I believe and confess that I am restored from curses into blessings. I trust and confess that I am restored from bondage into liberty.

I believe and confess that I have been restored from all oppression of wickedness to enjoy the fulness of redemption. I confess and pray back anything the devil has stolen from my marriage, ministry,

Church, business and nation. I pray for a hundred-fold restoration in every area of my life, in Jesus' mighty name, Amen.

PRAYER FOR CONCENTRATION

I pray that I will not be double-minded in any of my decisions. I will not lack focus nor lose concentration of my calling. I will enjoy maximum concentration in every godly plan I undertake for the progress of my life and destiny.

Nothing will distract my attention from my assignment and commission in life. I pray for a constant flow of supernatural concentration to pursue the reason for my existence on planet earth. I pray and confess that I will possess a very sharp and high level of concentration on the Word and the work of God.

I pray and confess that nothing, visible or invisible, will divert my attention from my God-given destiny. I believe and confess that my dreams and visions shall not be hindered nor thwarted.

My level of concentration in all my duties is unbeatable and unpredictable in the mighty name of Jesus and through the blood of the eternal covenant. Amen.

PRAYER FOR ABUNDANCE

I pray and confess that I will not lack abundance in life. I confess and believe that I will enjoy the fulness of the riches of abundance all the days of my life. I declare that every aspect of my life will receive a visitation of abundant grace, abundant peace and abundant joy.

I decree and declare over my life, good health in abundance. I refuse to lack in any good thing needed to make my dreams and vision a reality. I confess that God will supply all my needs according to His riches in glory through Christ Jesus, in all abundance; that I will never lack supply and support for the continuity of any good thing I have embarked upon. The blessings of the Lord will make me abundantly rich and I will lack nothing.

Now unto Him that is able to do exceedingly, abundantly above all that we ask or think according to the power that works in us, unto Jehovah be all the glory throughout the ages, in Jesus' name, Amen.

PRAYER FOR BLESSINGS

I declare that my going out and my coming in is blessed, and that anything I touch shall be blessed. I am a blessed person. I am blessed and highly favoured in all my ways by the Lord.

I confess that I am blessed with the gold of sheba. I will flourish like the glass of the earth. I believe and confess that the Lord has given me power to get wealth. My seed will never beg for bread. I confess that I will not borrow but give. My life will be a channel of blessings to many people in my generation.

I confess that I will flourish like a palm tree and I remain fresh in all my ways. The blessings of God upon my life will always make me rich on every side without the addition of sorrow. I will never lack any good thing.

I confess that I am blessed and no curse can work against my life. I confess that I am blessed in the morning, blessed in the evening, blessed every hour, blessed every minute. I confess that I am blessed every week and month of every year.

Blessed shall be the fruit of my body and all the works of my hands. The blessings of the Lord overtake me, my children, my spouse and my business. I confess that the blessings of God will follow me in life and eternity in the name of Jesus Christ, Amen.

PRAYER FOR BOLDNESS

I am a righteous man and am as bold as a lion. I pray and confess that I will not be moved by what I hear or see. I receive boldness over fear, intimidation and every threat of the wicked one.

I confess that I am seated with Christ Jesus in heavenly places, I therefore believe that I am bold like the Lion of the tribe of Judah. I confess that gloominess and thick darkness will not put fear in me to give up on my mission. I receive divine and supernatural boldness over principalities and powers.

I believe and accept that God has not given me the spirit of fear and timidity but of power, love and a sound mind of boldness.

By destiny, I believe that the Lord has empowered my tongue to boldly declare his word without any restriction or fear of people, both to the poor and rich. I confess that through boldness, I have overcome the enemy for good. By boldness, I confront every mountain before me. I command every mountain in my finances, in my family and in my ministry to become plain in Jesus' mighty name.

I am a redeemed child of God. I therefore take my rightful place in redemption, to stand before the throne of grace in boldness and to receive from God all that He has in store for me in Jesus' mighty name, Amen.

PRAYER FOR SENSITIVITY

I believe and confess that God has granted me supernatural sensitivity for foresight and insight. My mind is a brain-bank for creativity and divine inventions. I will not be overtaken by surprise at any satanic or human attack. I believe that God has given me a divine understanding of the times and seasons that we live in.

I pray that God will make me sensitive to every invisible device of satan aimed at my life and destiny. I believe that my mind has been quickened and empowered. I have the mind of Christ. The gift of the Spirit is at work in me. I can discern every spirit that comes my way, including every demon that disguises as an angel of light.

I will never be taken off-guard by any situation in life. God opens my mind to have a pre-knowledge of any move that is contrary to the promotions and blessings of God for my life. Through sensitivity, the Holy Ghost shall have His way in my life, in Jesus' name, Amen.

PRAYER FOR MARRIAGE

I release myself from any demonic union in the spirit. As a virtuous woman/faithful man I refuse to be single. I am delivered from the spirit of singleness. I bind any satanic power from my family line that is holding back my marital miracle. The anointing of the Holy Ghost makes my face shine and increases my physical beauty; it makes me attractive to my marital partner.

In the name of Jesus, I claim all the qualities of a godly and faithful person. The Spirit of the Lord overshadows me with fresh glory as a child of God. I am protected and hidden in the Blood of Jesus from spiritual partners.

I call forth my husband/wife in the name of Jesus. Whoever he/she is, I pray that the wind of the Holy Spirit will blow him/her to my direction in the name of Jesus. I pray and establish this in Jesus' mighty name.

PRAYER FOR FRUITFULNESS

Children are my heritage in the Lord. I possess all my children in the name of Jesus. I confess that barrenness is not my protion because I am a fruitful vine, created to increase and multiply.

I pray and confess that the fruit of my body shall not be destroyed. I refuse to be barren in the name of Jesus. I wash my womb in the Blood of the Lamb. I humiliate and overcome the spirit of miscarriage in the name of Jesus.

I confess that the Holy Spirit strengthens my inner being, my physical body and my biological systems, to enable me to carry my miracle seed. Thank you Lord for the fruit of the womb. Thank you for making me the mother of many through the work of the Holy Spirit.

I believe and confess that I am no more under the power of sorrow and rejection. I am grateful to God for putting laughter in my mouth. May the name of the Lord be praised for making me a fruitful woman.

PRAYER FOR HOLINESS

Dignity is rooted in holiness. Dignity is my portion in life because I operate in holiness and righteousness. I destroy the grip of sin over my life. I choose to be holy because I serve a holy God. In the name of Jesus I depart from iniquity because I call upon the name of the Lord and He knows me. The blood of Jesus has sanctified and purified me from all the works of the flesh, in Jesus' name.

I bind the spirit of fornication and destroy its influence over my life. I loose myself by the power of the Holy Spirit. I destroy the power of greed, lust of the flesh, lust of the eyes and the love of money in the name of Jesus. I stop you Satan in the name of Jesus, you will no more have authority over my emotions. I will wait for the appointed time of marriage. I will no more be a victim of the trap of pre-marital sex, abortion or any kind of immorality. The blood of Jesus sets me free and cleanses me from every guilt of sin and immorality.

I believe and confess that I am the beauty of the Lord because I have made my choice for righteousness and holiness. I am a golden vessel. Jesus makes me shine everyday in holiness and righteousness by the power of His Spirit.

I confess that the Lord has delivered me from the powers of darkness and has empowered me to serve Him in holiness and righteousness all the days of my life. Thank you Lord Jesus, Amen.

PRAYER FOR WISDOM

I believe and confess that I have received the Spirit of wisdom and understanding from God. I have overcome the spirit of dullness in Jesus' name.

The Lord Jesus has enlarged my thought pattern and granted me the Spirit of counsel, the Spirit of knowledge and of the fear of the Lord. I am overshadowed with the Spirit of the Lord.

I claim a creative mind to make things happen to the glory of God. I claim wisdom for my business, marriage and life in general. I embrace the Wisdom of Solomon to operate with supernatural intelligence, in Jesus' name.

The Lord will supply me with wisdom on how to handle people. I receive wisdom for wise decision-making. I receive wisdom for my choices in life. I choose to be wise because I serve a God of wisdom who created the whole world by his unfathomable wisdom.

Through wisdom my destiny is built. Through understanding it is established. And through knowledge it is filled with every imaginable good thing, in Jesus' name.

PRAYER FOR SUCCESS

I choose to succeed in the name of Jesus. I confess that success is my portion in life. Failure will no more have authority over my business, my marriage and all my programmes in life. I destroy the spirit of failure and shame in the name of Jesus. The Lord is on my side to succeed.

I believe and confess that Jesus has changed my destiny from failure to success. Therefore the spirit of failure has no access into my life. My dreams and vision in life shall succeed. My business shall succeed. My marriage and my entire family shall succeed in the mighty name of Jesus.

I choose to succeed in everything I do in this life. I pray and confess that the Lord Jesus will make a way for me to be a winner and not a loser. I see beyond my present situation in Jesus' name, because the Lord is committed to my success in life.

PRAYER FOR ACCOMPLISHMENT

I believe and confess that I shall not die but live to witness the completion of every project I undertake in this life. I pray for and receive the grace for accomplishment. I will surely finish all that I start to do in Jesus' name.

I receive divine provision for the completion of my building projects. I receive supernatural grace for the completion of my financial projects. I pray and confess that the God of heaven will make a way for me where there seems to be no way and make every impossible situation possible in the name of Jesus.

I receive finishing power in the name of Jesus. The Lord will anoint my hands for battle. He will strengthen my hands for work. The same hands that began the work will be anointed by the power of the Holy Spirit for unqestionabe accomplishment.

My God will strengthen me to accomplish all my projects with distinction in the name of Jesus. Any distraction from the devil will not succeed against me in the name of Jesus. That which God has started in me shall be brought to completion in Jesus' mighty name, Amen.

PRAYER FOR HEALING

I receive my healing in the name of Jesus. By the power of the blood of Jesus, every sickness in my life is destroyed never to come back again.

I believe and confess that the blood of Jesus separates me from the spirit of blood cancer, asthma, fibroids and hypertension. The anointing of God destroys every yoke of sickness upon my life. Every disease in my life comes to an end in Jesus' name. I refuse to be sick. I choose to be healed and stay healed in Jesus' mighty name.

I pray and believe that the blood of Jesus sets me free from sickness. By the stripes of the Lord Jesus Christ, I am already made whole. I claim my liberty by the anointing of the Holy Spirit and by the authority of God's Word. I am forever free from sickness and disease. I am healed by the blood of the Lamb.

PRAYER FOR JOY

I believe and confess that this is the day the Lord has made, therefore, I will rejoice and be glad in it. Joy is my birthright. It is the fruit of the Holy Ghost in me.

I destroy the spirit of heaviness that is out to rob me of my joy. Satan, lift up your hands from my happiness. I resist and overpower you in the name of Jesus. The joy of the Lord is my strength. Joy is my portion in life.

My destiny will not be destroyed by the spirit of heaviness in the name of Jesus. There is no more room for unhappiness in my life. From henceforth, everyday of my life will be a day of joy. The word of the Lord shall be the theme of my song all day long. My heart is filled with joyful melodies to the glory of God. Even upon my bed I shall sing God's praise. No man will take my joy away from me today in Jesus' name.

PRAYER FOR RECOVERY

I confess and believe that I have totally recovered from every satanic attack. I claim total recovery of my health, finance and every lost anointing and gift. I confess and claim recovery from fear, failure, wounds, pain, sorrow, disapointments and frustration in Jesus' name.

I may have failed in business, but by the power of God I choose to rise again. Because the Spirit of God dwells in me, my physical body is quickened and restored back to life. I recover everything the devil has stolen from me.

SECTION THREE:

THE REASON FOR POSITIVE CONFESSION

THE REASON FOR POSITIVE CONFESSION

There are many other prayer needs you can pray this way. My primary purpose for teaching you this type of confession prayer is for you to know how to lay claim on every provision Jesus made for you at calvary.

Positive confession prayer is what I call "prayer made simple". You can pray without sweat when you learn to pray positively with the Word of God.

You do not need to be saved for many years to pray this way. I have heard Christians complain that they do not pray because they know not how to organise themselves in prayer. I do not believe in this kind of talk. This is why I have written this book. I have committed to you a very easy way of praying without having to know all the scriptures.

As you work on yourself and upgrade your knowledge of the Word of God, you

will know how to lay hold of the promises God has made available to you through positive and powerful prayer.

Positive confession prayer will shape your mentality for breakthroughs, for out of the abundance of the heart the mouth speaks. When you think success, you will confess and pray success. It is time believers move to the breakthrough level through positive confession.

"DEATH AND LIFE ARE IN THE POWER OF THE TONGUE, AND THEY THAT LOVE IT SHALL EAT THE FRUIT THEREOF"

(PROVERBS 18:21)

Whatever comes out of your mouth matters, even when you think you are just joking and you do not mean what you are saying.

You do not need to get knocked down by a car to die. The easiest way to destruction is through negative confessions of the mouth.

Whenever you confess negative things with your mouth, remember that all you are saying is what you love and desire to see. Your wish will be granted, exactly how you confess it.

Your confession is like a seed you have planted. Be sure that you will eat of the fruit of your confessions.

"A MAN SHALL BE SATISFIED WITH GOOD BY THE FRUIT OF HIS MOUTH"

(PROVERBS 12:14)

Friend, when you make positive confessions, you reap blessings and not curses. Many Christians are running from place to place for deliverance. Even though I believe in deliverance, I also believe that most of our problems are self- inflicted.

Deliver yourself from self-inflicted curses by speaking and praying the Word of God into every situation of your life. Begin to enforce the efficiency of God's Word into your life for total recovery through positive confession prayer.

You will not die but live long because all it takes for you to enjoy a long life is embodied in your tongue - this is the power of your confessions. Train your mouth to feed your life with blessings through positive confessions. Let your mouth feed your business, your marriage and every concerned area of your life with positive confessions. Your mouth is a miracle bank connecting you to the riches and resources of heaven.

FINAL WORD:
BE STRONG

There is an end-time battle going on. It is not for weak vessels. Prayerless Christians cannot survive the heat of this battle. It is often said, and I agree, that a prayerful Christian is a powerful Christian; a prayerless Christian is a powerless Christian. The choice is yours to make between victory and defeat.

"BUT THE PEOPLE THAT DO KNOW THERE GOD SHALL BE STRONG, AND DO EXPLOITS"

(DANIEL 11:32B)

Power for exploits and accomplishment in life belongs to the people that know their God. This knowledge of God comes through fellowship with the Son, Jesus Christ, and by the Holy Spirit. The deeper your fellowship with God, the stronger you become.

I encourage you to daily develop your

relationship with God so that you can be strong in every dimension of your life—financially, physically, matrimonially, emotionally and spiritually.

"BUT THEY THAT WAIT UPON THE LORD SHALL RENEW THEIR STRENGTH"

(ISAIAH 40:31)

Step out of your comfort zone. Stop grieving over your problems. Get into the secret place of the Lord Almighty where your strength will be renewed. As you encounter God in prayer, you will dominate every circumstance around you.

Do not underestimate the strength of God in you. Even in your weakness, treasure the "little" strength that you have and the Lord will lift you to your rightful position of power.

"LET THE WEAK SAY, 'I AM STRONG'"

(JOEL 3:10B)

ABOUT THE AUTHOR

James Osborn Nanjo is an end-time, fire-brand prophetic Evangelist with a heavenly calling to reach out to the end-time generation with the gospel of Jesus Christ. As a travelling messenger, he teaches and preaches the word of God with signs and wonders following. He is also a regular speaker at prophetic gatherings, revival meetings, conferences and crusades. His radio ministry, Voice of Redemption, (98.2 FM) in the city of London, has impacted thousands of people from different backgrounds and cultures, with amazing testimonies of the power of God.

As the leader of *World Restoration Ministries*, James Osborn Nanjo also serves as an associate of *Ampiah Kwofi World Outreach* of *Global Revival Ministries*.

The ministry of this young man encourages people to rise up to their godly heritage and divine destiny through prayer revivals, breaking all cultural barriers and reaching the world with the mandate of the Great Commission.

TO CONTACT JAMES OSBORN NANJO, WRITE:

World Restoration Ministries
18 Milton Court Road
London SE14 6JL
Tel: 020 8692 6192/07939 276568
Email: osborjnwrm@hotmail.com
(Please include your prayer request and comments when you write).

For additional copies of this book or any enquiry, please contact the address above.

In USA, please contact:

World Restoration Partners
2731 Tennyson Belv'd
Columbus Ohio 43232
Tel: (+1) 614 8569053

In Ghana, please contact:

Global Revival Ministries
PO Box 12219
Accra North
Ghana
Tel: (+233) 921 407938